The Carn

The Complete Carnivore Diet Guide For Beginners

Introduction

If anyone could come up with a diet for people who hate diets, know the dangers of vegetables or just hate them for whatever reason, it would be the carnivore diet in which you're supposed to subsist on meat and animal products alone.

As that sinks in, I would totally understand if you made a reaction like "oh no, that's impossible!" because for one, we've been taught to eat vegetables since we were young- as the only way to be strong and healthy.

Most of us cannot imagine a life without fruits and vegetables, which is fine before truly understanding what this is all about. Wouldn't it be tragic to finally learn that animal foods are all we need to be healthy and that veggies are actually detrimental to our health? Perhaps a huge direct punch in the face to all we've learnt in school and all the health headlines and nutrition in the media everywhere?

Indeed, the carnivore diet does seem like the most radical trend that bucks conventional nutritional guidelines and advice. After all, we know that meat is dangerous, particularly when you eat huge amounts of it, right?

I'm sorry for this spoiler alert but history and science itself has revealed that eating meat and animal products

The Carnivore Diet

is actually healthy- and vegetables, though good at face value, cause harm to us in ways few of us actually know.

But hey, don't worry; this book is here to provide all the information you need to understand why this is so, and introduce you properly to the carnivore diet.

All you need to keep in mind as you read this book is that the carnivore diet has become a hot eating trend for a very good reason. Many people have reported multiple significant benefits from taking up an all-meat diet. Some of these benefits include quicker weight loss, better mental clarity, improved energy and athletic performance, and healthier digestion. All these and more will be discussed in detail in this book.

Better keep your eyes peeled for some really good recipes (to get you started in the best way possible) somewhere in the course of the book!

Let's begin!

Table of Contents

Introduction _____ 2

What Is The Carnivore Diet? _____ 8

    The Past And Present Meat Mongers _____ 8

    The Dangers Of Plants That Nobody Talks About 11

The Benefits Of The Carnivore Diet _____ 17

Eat This Not That _____ 23

    What To Eat & What Not To Eat _____ 23

Breakfast Recipes _____ 26

    Steak And Eggs Breakfast _____ 26

    Eggs, Ground Beef & Cheese Breakfast Casserole _____ 28

    Zero Carb Pancakes _____ 30

    Pork, Egg and Shrimp "Pancakes" _____ 31

    Cheat's Eggs Benedict _____ 33

    Meat Lovers Breakfast Skillet _____ 35

    Basic Eggs in Broth_____ 38

    'Baked Egg Carnivore Custard' _____ 39

    Sausage Breakfast Sandwich _____ 41

Ham & Cheese Egg Cups _____ 43

Butter Coffee _____ 45

No-Bread Keto Breakfast Sandwich _____ 46

Ham And Swiss Omelet _____ 48

Breakfast Pockets _____ 50

Lunch Recipes _____ **52**

The Best Garlic Cilantro Salmon _____ 52

Skillet Rib Eye Steaks _____ 54

Olive Oil-Basted Grass-Fed Strip Steak _____ 56

Vivica's Keto Roast Chicken _____ 58

Grilled Split Lobster _____ 60

Grilled Shrimp Seasoning _____ 62

Duck Leg Confit _____ 64

Beef (Heart) Steak _____ 66

Grilled Beef Liver _____ 68

Moroccan Liver Kebabs _____ 70

Fresh Oysters _____ 73

Grilled Lamb Chops _____ 75

AIP Bacon-Wrapped Salmon _____ 77

Dinner Recipes _____ 78

Baked Chicken Breast _____ 78

Pressure Cooked Pork Loin Roast _____ 80

Crispy Oven Roasted Salmon _____ 82

Pinchos De Pollo _____ 83

Whole Roasted Beef Tenderloin _____ 85

Coconut-Lime Skirt Steak _____ 87

Philly Cheese Steak Casserole _____ 89

Mini Cheeseburger Meatloaves _____ 91

Grilled Marinated Venison Steak _____ 93

Crockpot Venison BBQ _____ 95

Smoked Duck or Goose _____ 96

Keto Pizza _____ 97

Snack/Appetizer/Dessert Recipes _____ 99

Honey Sriracha Lime Duck Legs _____ 99

Elk Burgers _____ 101

Papa's Duck Poppers _____ 102

Ham Pizza Snacks _____ 104

Pizza Cup Snacks _____ 105

Tangy Barbecue Wings _____ 106

Pork Satay _____ 108

Tavuk Göğsü _____ 110

Lattice Mincemeat Dessert Tart _____ 112

Conclusion _____ **114**

Quoted Studies _____ **115**

What Is The Carnivore Diet?

As you already know, the carnivore diet is a diet in which you only eat animal foods like meat and products like eggs and milk. Every other food is severely restricted. That means no vegetables, no fruits, and especially, no carbs. You can think of it as the total opposite of a vegan diet.

According to proponents and enthusiasts of this diet, plant foods are not essential to us, and that carbohydrate, which is found in plants, is the only macronutrient that's non-essential. That means that our bodies mainly require fats and proteins to thrive.

This diet is also very straightforward and simple because you don't do things like food timing, portion control, calorie counting and other things that you'd typically do on a regular diet.

The Past And Present Meat Mongers

To the best of my knowledge, earth hasn't yet produced a civilization that has successfully eaten a pure vegan diet from birth through death, whereas, throughout recorded history, there are many examples of people from various geographical, cultural and ethnic backgrounds who have managed to live on diets that are mainly composed of meats for decades, generations and lifetimes.

The Carnivore Diet

Before I mention a few of the ones I have in mind, you first have to note that our ancestors survived on a diet that was meat-based. Yes, all the wild fruit, leaves and roots were not energy efficient for them, leave alone enough to help them get by in the harsh preexisting environmental conditions.

As a result, they had to hunt game, consume animal products thus, according to proponents of the carnivore diet, the human body has evolved to optimally run on a meat-based diet.

Today, there are examples of real people who are still thriving on mostly-meat diets as they have for decades.

Let me mention a few of them:

- The Inuit who live in the Canadian Arctic live on seal, fish, whale meat and walrus.

- The Steppe nomads of Mongolia thrive on mostly meat and dairy products.

- The Chukotka living in the Russian Arctic thrive on marine animals, meat and fish.

- The Masaai warriors of East Africa live on diets that mainly comprise milk, blood and meat.

- The Brazilian Gauchos have been nourishing themselves with beef

- The Sioux of South Dakota have been enjoying a diet of Buffalo meat.

There are two things you need to note here:

If you look at the arctic, for instance, there are no vegetables and fruits (perhaps with an exception of summer, when there would be few, young willow shoots and some bits of green, which would be used as relish to meats and a few berries), which means that throughout the year, most of its inhabitants actually consume close to zero fruits and vegetables. There is zero fiber in seal or fish, or in an arctic bird.

Secondly, these people are some of the healthiest people in the world; some of them live in some of the harshest environments in the world and still live longer than most of us who live in near-perfect societies.

More than four decades ago, the region of Point Hope, Alaska, where people were still eating mostly meat (since the area was pretty isolated) became a subject of a research study that was published back in 1972. The researchers found that inhabitants of Point Hope recorded a low incidence of heart disease; actually, it was ten times lower than that in the overall US Caucasian population.

More specifically, their triglyceride (fat in the bloodstream) levels were about 85 mg/dl compared to the standard U.S triglyceride levels which, at the time averaged over 100mg/dl:

So, who are you not to eat meat?

Not convinced? Let's continue.

We'll take a look at the potential benefits of eating meat and animal products alone -but before that, let me explain to you why plants are dangerous.

The Dangers Of Plants That Nobody Talks About

Plants can harm us in many ways, but one of the most pronounced ways they try to keep us from eating them are what scientists call anti-nutrients.

Anti-nutrients are chemical compounds found in plants that, when ingested, interfere with the absorption of important minerals and nutrients. They thus keep your body from being an efficient micronutrient sponge that it was designed to be.

Animals and human beings usually pull the nourishment we require from our surroundings but with evolution, plants have developed their ability to fight back. Anti-nutrients or what most people refer to as nutrient-sapping phytochemicals, protect the plants from being eaten to the point of becoming extinct. Anti-nutrients are most concentrated in legumes like beans, grains, nuts and in different roots, leaves and fruits.

Let's take a look at a few examples.

Lectins

Lectins are proteins that stick to the intestinal wall and lead to intestinal permeability, thus causing problems in the digestive system. When you eat food, it moves through your gastrointestinal tract, bangs into the lining of your gut and causes a micro-trauma. Under normal circumstances, your cells repair these bruises and bumps before it becomes a serious issue. Unfortunately, lectins come in to make the process worse by sticking to the walls of your gut and preventing any repair. The resulting damage leads to some inflammation in your tract.

Now imagine a situation where you are eating a lot of lectins; your gut wall would develop holes and its contents would then enter your bloodstream, leading to leaky gut syndrome.

There are literally thousands of lectin varieties, and they are found in most plant species. However, the most common sources of lectins are nightshade vegetables, legumes and grains. These plants usually have more lectins than other food sources (which also contain the chemical) like nuts, potatoes, tomatoes, eggplants and wheat.

If you experience stomach problems, migraines, brain fog, acne, joint pain and inflammation, you might be having a problem with lectins. I however need to mention that in nightshades, lectins are a common autoimmune trigger and tend to cause sensitivities in many people.

Phytic acid/ phytate

Phytic acid is one of the most harmful anti-nutrients in plants. It blocks the absorption of minerals like iron, calcium, zinc and magnesium in the body. This chemical is found in nuts, whole grains, seeds and legumes like soybeans.

What phytic acid does is that it binds to these minerals and prevents their absorption such that in the end, your body gets very little nutrition from food.

What's more; phytic acid inhibits digestive enzymes which include amylase, trypsin and pepsin. Pepsin and trypsin break down protein while amylase is needed for the breakdown of starch. When you don't have these enzymes in the right amounts, food won't be processed well in your body- which means that you'll be getting very little of the key nutrients.

Your body requires enough muscle to burn fat and to build muscle, your body requires enough protein. Nonetheless, the amount of protein you get from food largely depends on how healthy your gut is. Read on to see how the other anti-nutrients and the carnivore diet affect the gut's health.

Oxalic acid/oxalate

If you're a lover of kale and spinach, you may have to look for other friends because they may be causing more harm than good to your body. Oxalic acid is a compound that's found in many plants such as cruciferous vegetables, which include broccoli, radishes, kale and cauliflower. It is also found in chard, beets, spinach, black pepper, parsley, beans, berries, nuts and chocolate.

What does oxylic acid do?

Oxalic acid usually binds to calcium in your blood to form sharp crystals, which are small enough to be deposited anywhere in the body. In the end, they lead to muscle pain or even kidney stones if they're deposited in the kidneys.

Oxalates also lead to a condition in women known as vulvodynia; this problem translates to painful sex when the oxalic acid crystals are deposited in the labia.

If you're particularly sensitive to this chemical, all you need is a small amount of oxalic acid to experience uncomfortable burning in the throat, eyes, mouth and ears. When you take large amounts of this compound, you are likely to experience muscle weakness, nausea, diarrhea and abdominal pain.

Gluten

Gluten is a kind of protein found in barley, oats, rye and wheat that leads to intestinal permeability also known as leaky gut. The issue with gluten is that human beings are not able to digest it, which means that it's generally impossible to benefit from the gluten proteins found in all foods containing gluten.

An indigestible substance in the body or digestive system usually causes an immune response. These immune responses usually take the form of inflammation, and inflammation is usually the cause of digestive discomfort, brain fog and inadequate absorption of nutrients.

Unfortunately, grains that contain gluten are highly addictive. This is because when these grains break down in the gut, compounds known as gluteomorphins are produced, and they usually trigger the same brain receptors as heroin and other opiate drugs.

Other anti-nutrients include the following:

Saponins

Saponins are usually found in legumes. The name of this anti-nutrient comes from the ability of this anti-nutrient to form soap-like foams when it gets into a solution. Just like lectins, saponins tend bind to the gut and increase intestinal permeability.

Tannins

I'm sure you've heard of tannins- the compound that affords wine its dry taste. Tannins are polyphenols that occur naturally in different plants- in their seeds, leaves, bark, fruit skins and wood.

What you may not know is that tannins are harmful to the body because they prevent your body from absorbing iron from food, which can lead to anemia.

Trypsin inhibitors

Trypsin inhibitors are a kind of proteins that inhibit the activity of an enzyme in the body known as trypsin. Trypsin is one of the digestive enzymes that helps in the digestion and absorption of protein. When you consume trypsin regularly, your body stops benefiting from the protein in the food you take.

That said, let's explore some of the benefits of the carnivore diet.

Now that you know possible dangers of plant based foods, the next question you might be asking is; so what makes animals based foods any better? Let's discuss some of the benefits of a carnivore diet next.

The Benefits Of The Carnivore Diet

Boosts the cognitive function

According to one study conducted on healthy men, boosting your intake of meat protein and reducing carbohydrate intake improves reaction time, which may help in boosting perception and focus.

Secondly, red meat in particular increases the branched-chain amino acids (BCAA) as well as a chemical known as phenylalanine in the blood. The former (BCAA) helps in reducing fatigue and the latter is a precursor to norepinephrine and dopamine hormones, which regulate mood and stress.

Third, according to the Chinese study below, children who consume meat regularly are likely to maintain their cognitive function when they grow older. Similarly, Korean teenagers and children who consumed more meat and poultry recorded higher scores on cognitive tests.

There was another study that investigated the correlation between dementia and diet in some parts of China. This study found that two dietary patterns were associated with lower rates of cognitive decline in older people: one of them was based on vegetables, fruits and the other was based on soy and meat. Vegetables and fruits were clearly seen to carry a higher risk factor than meat.

Lastly, the carnivore diet helps people with obsessive compulsive disorder (OCD) by relieving the condition's symptoms. As a victim of OCD, you tend to have very high amounts of a neurotransmitter known as glutamate. When this neurotransmitter is overactive in the brain, it tends to cause neurological disorders and increases your sensitivity to pain.

Delicious foods like soy sauce and parmesan cheese usually contain high levels of glutamate. Plant proteins actually have as high as 40% glutamate, while the animal proteins have 11-22%. You also have to note that glutamate is also added to food as MSG or monosodium glutamate.

Thankfully, the carnivore diet doesn't condone canned foods or those with any kind of additives.

According to these studies, it's clear that carnivore diets can assist in restricting dietary glutamate, as long as canned meat, preserved seafood or processed meat are not included on their food lists.

While there's very little dietary glutamate that reaches the brain, studies show that any diet that restricts glutamate goes a long way in helping people with OCD. In one case study, a person suffering from OCD experienced a significant improvement on a glutamate-restricted diet; his symptoms however returned as a result of MSG.

Helps with autoimmunity

As you may already know, people experience autoimmunity when they take foods like wheat, eggs proteins and milk. What happens is that the antibodies meant to protect you from infection react against these proteins (which your immune system perceives to be unknown triggers); they attack your own brain tissues, leading to brain fog and other neurological issues.

Meat contains a lot of zinc. This mineral usually increases regulatory cells known as T cells, thus preventing autoimmunity. You need to note that zinc supplements have been able to improve symptoms in some people with autism, a condition that is heavily linked with autoimmunity:

Meat also contains high amounts of B vitamins, which tend to improve lupus symptoms, which is an autoimmune condition. One of these vitamins is B6, which has been seen to have the capacity to suppress inflammation and support immune function in people suffering from lupus.

Improves heart health

Saturated fats (which meat contains in high amounts) have for a long time been believed to be a risk factor for heart health until recently -in 2015, when a meta-analysis proved that there is no correlation between cardiovascular disease and saturated fat intake.

Diets high in fat (which includes saturated fat) have been seen to be effective in lowering cholesterol and triglycerides in the body, as well as reducing blood pressure. Researchers conducted multiple studies on obese people and saw that a high fat diet is able to reduce the bad cholesterol that clogs arteries (low density lipoprotein), triglycerides and glucose in the blood, and increases the good cholesterol (high density lipoprotein).

Such diets also alter the structure of the LDL molecules, increasing the size of the particles. These bigger particles are generally less likely to produce plaques.

All these benefits are great for your heart, which makes the carnivore diet ideal when you want to improve your heart health.

It improves your gut

The food you eat highly determines the type of bacteria that lives in your intestines. When you eat plants, you get a lot of fiber from them, and that promotes the growth of bacteria that processes the carbohydrates into short-chain fatty acids. On the other hand, consuming the carnivore diet (high animal fat and protein) reduces the overall population of the gut bacteria and boosts the population of clostridia and bacteroides.

When you have low levels of bacteroids, you are more likely to develop inflammatory bowel diseases such as ulcerative colitis and Crohn's disease. This suggests if you are currently suffering from inflammatory bowel disease, consuming more meat would help you manage it.

Lastly, beef has been seen to have high amounts of an amino acid known as glutamine. This compound protects the tight junctions of the intestinal wall and has the ability to protect you from leaky gut.

Glutamine also helps people with irritable bowel syndrome improve their symptoms. In one study, taking 15g of glutamine per day for 8 weeks helped people with IBS by reducing diarrhea.

Helps in weight loss

Many studies have confirmed that people on a low carbohydrate diet lose weight a lot faster than most weight loss diets. These studies show that people on a low carb, high fat diet lost more weight than people on low fat diets:

Since the mid-1800s, low carb diets have been a weight loss strategy and one of the reasons they work is that they reduce the production of insulin (the sugar and fat storage hormone).

When you reduce sugar intake, you automatically reduce its storage, and the subsequent fat storage that occurs when the sugar/glucose stores (glycogen) are full. This also promotes weight loss because the body starts burning fat since the amount of glucose (which it normally uses as fuel) is low in the body.

According to some studies, low carb diets also boost the amount of energy your body burns by about 300 calories if you consume the same amount of calories- even though this result has not been adequately confirmed.

Another factor is added sugar. Most processed foods usually have refined sugars added during their production. These sugars promote weight gain and metabolic disease. A true carnivore diet doesn't contain any sugar, which totally helps in avoiding this risk.

Lastly, protein increases satiety. In other words, it enable you to feel as though you've had enough food, and that feeling lingers for longer than when you've consumed carbohydrates. In the long run, you consume fewer calories. A high-protein diet has been shown to boost a better body composition and promote weight loss. I don't think there's a diet that contains more protein than the carnivore diet.

So what exactly do you eat while on the carnivore diet and what should you avoid? Let's discuss that next.

Eat This Not That

What To Eat & What Not To Eat

A meat-only diet is quite self-explanatory- all you'll be eating is meat. However, just like all diets, this one has some gray areas.

The foods you can eat on this diet include the following:

Red meat- including beef, lamb and pork; while making emphasis on fattier meat cuts to take in sufficient calories. The other options you have include the following:

- Water
- Salt and pepper
- Poultry
- Organ meats
- Lard
- Fish
- Eggs
- Butter
- Bone marrow
- Bone broth

There are foods that are considered "okay" on this diet. These foods are generally acceptable as some people argue that they come from animals. They include the following:

- Milk

- Cheese

- Yogurt

Others

- Coffee

- Tea

- Healthy condiments and seasonings are also allowed.

Foods Not Allowed on the Carnivore Diet

- Vegetables including legumes

- Pasta

- Fruits

- Seeds

- Nuts

- Grains

- Alcohol

The Carnivore Diet

Let's now put what we've learned about the diet into perspective by discussing some delicious recipes you can prepare while on the carnivore diet.

Breakfast Recipes

Steak And Eggs Breakfast

Serves 1

Ingredients

Chuck eye steak, 6 ounces 1/2 inch thick

1/4 teaspoon freshly ground black pepper, divided

2 large eggs

1 tablespoon chopped parsley for garnish, optional

1/4 teaspoon kosher salt, divided

Avocado oil spray

Pinch red pepper flakes

Directions

Preheat the grill. Get the steak out of the fridge and season it with a pinch of black pepper and salt.

Spray the grill using oil and grill the steak for two minutes on each side for medium-rare; if you're using a dual contact grill, aim for 3 minutes in total.

As the steak cooks, set a nonstick skillet over medium heat and heat it for about four minutes. When the steak is finished cooking, transfer it to a plate and cover it with foil loosely and let it rest.

In the meantime, prepare the eggs. Spray the skillet with oil and break the eggs into the skillet set over medium heat. Fry them for about five minutes, or until the whites are ready.

Now put the cooked eggs on a plate and season them with a pinch of pepper and salt. Season the eggs and steak with red pepper flakes and garnish with chopped parsley; dig in!

Eggs, Ground Beef & Cheese Breakfast Casserole

Serves 12

Ingredients

1 pound lean ground beef, or turkey

2 teaspoons dried sage

1 1/4 teaspoons salt, divided

1/2 teaspoon onion powder

Pinch of crushed red pepper flakes

6 ounces (about 1 1/2 cups) grated cheddar cheese

1 1/2 cups milk

1 tablespoon brown sugar

1 1/2 teaspoons dried basil

1/2 teaspoon garlic powder

1/4 teaspoon marjoram

Freshly ground black pepper, to taste

8 eggs

1 teaspoon ground mustard powder

Directions

The Carnivore Diet

Put your oven rack in the middle area of your oven and preheat it to 350 degrees F. Grease or coat your 9 x 13 inch baking dish with cooking spray.

Set a Dutch oven, pot, pan or large skillet over medium-high heat and then add the ground beef. Cook it until all the pink disappears, breaking it apart and stirring until the beef cooks.

Add the sage, sugar, ¾ teaspoon of salt, basil, onion powder, red pepper flakes, marjoram, garlic powder, black pepper and brown sugar to a bowl and mix well until combined, set aside.

When the meat is ready, drain the grease from the skillet and add in the spice blend while stirring. Remove the skillet from the heat and let it cool for a couple of minutes.

Spread the meat in the prepared baking dish and sprinkle the meat with grated cheddar. Add the eggs, mustard powder, milk, ground pepper and ½ teaspoon of salt to a large bowl and whisk well to combine.

Pour the egg mixture over the cheese/beef mixture in the dish evenly and bake for between 50 and 55 minutes, until the eggs are golden brown and nicely puffed, and the middle is set. Let it sit for five minutes before you slice and serve.

Note:

You can bake half of this recipe in an 8 x 8 inch square dish and check for doneness after a period of 40 minutes.

Zero Carb Pancakes

Serves 1-2

Ingredients

2 ounces cream cheese

2 eggs

Directions

Let the cream cheese soften before you blend, and blend using a food processor until smooth.

Add to a hot pan and cook just like ordinary pancakes, flipping when you see the batter bubbling in the pan.

Enjoy!

Pork, Egg and Shrimp "Pancakes"

Serves 4-5

Ingredients

3/4 pound ground pork

2 or 3 minced garlic cloves

3 green onion, chopped

1/8 pound of mung bean thread noodles (make sure to soak them in hot water for about 10 minutes and drain them)

1/4 pound raw, chopped (very fine to almost a ground consistency) shrimp

6 eggs

1/3 cup dried wood ear mushroom strips, soaked in hot water for 10 minutes, and drained

2 or 3 chopped shallots

Cracked black pepper

6-7 healthy dashes of nuoc mam

1 teaspoon sugar

Directions

Add the eggs to a bowl and beat them well. Add the rest of the ingredients to a large, separate mixing bowl and combine.

Add in the eggs over the meat mixture and mix everything together using your hands until well integrated.

Oil a non-stick pan and heat it up. Pour the batter on the pan, cover and cook over medium-low heat for five minutes.

Flip and repeat the process, uncovered.

Serve and enjoy!

Cheat's Eggs Benedict

Serves 1

Ingredients

1 large egg

½ teaspoon salt

2 tablespoons Hollandaise sauce from a jar

2 teaspoons white vinegar

1½ ounces ham steak

Black pepper

Directions

Add the egg into a ramekin and set aside.

Pour one inch of water to a sauce pan then add the vinegar and season with salt generously. Let the water simmer and using a spoon handle, swirl the water round gently in one direction.

As the water swirls, add the egg into the middle of the swirl. Turn the heat off and cover. Leave it to do its thing for about five minutes.

As the egg cooks, warm the ham steak for about 2 minutes on every side on a grill pan.

The Carnivore Diet

Place the ham on a plate, and then use a slotted spoon to remove the freshly cooked egg from the water. Pour over a bit of the Hollandaise sauce, then season it with black pepper and enjoy!

Meat Lovers Breakfast Skillet

Serves 8

Ingredients

1 pound Wright smoked bacon, cut into 1-inch pieces, plus more whole bacon strips to serve

6 ounces cured chorizo, diced

1 cup bell pepper, diced (I used red and green)

8 large eggs

1 teaspoon salt

2 cups shredded cheddar cheese

6 ounces ham, diced

1 cup yellow onion, diced

2 green onions, sliced

1 cup milk (I used whole milk)

1/2 teaspoon black pepper

Directions

Heat your oven to 400 degrees F.

Prepare the bacon in a large skillet set over medium heat, stirring occasionally until crisp. Grab a slotted spoon and transfer the bacon to a plate, set aside.

Now add the chorizo and ham to the same skillet and cook for 3-4 minutes, or until it turns light brown then transfer to a plate using a slotted spoon and set aside.

Add the bell peppers, onion and green onion to the pan drippings in the skillet you've been using and sauté those ingredients until soft and fragrant, for four minutes. Turn off the heat and allow the dish to cool for a short while.

Beat the eggs thoroughly in a separate bowl and add in the milk while whisking. Add the black pepper and salt and then add in the bacon, chorizo, ham and the pepper-onion mixture as you stir. Pour the mixture into the skillet and cover using a foil.

Bake until the eggs are well set and cooked through, for about 40 -45 minutes. Uncover and cook for 3-5 minutes until they're slightly golden.

Serve the fish immediately with a couple more whole bacon strips if you want.

Note:

The meat lovers' breakfast skillet is best made the night before; cover and store in your fridge to bake in the morning.

The Carnivore Diet

Lastly, you're free to adjust the quantities of the meat to suit your family's preference.

Basic Eggs in Broth

Ingredients

1-2 cups broth of choice – like chicken, fish, beef or pork

Grated parmesan cheese

Salt and pepper, to taste

1-2 eggs

Several sprigs parsley, chopped

Directions

Bring the broth to a simmer and then add in the eggs.

Simmer for a couple of minutes until the egg whites cook, but the yolks are still soft and runny.

Top with parsley, parmesan cheese, pepper and salt, to taste.

Enjoy!

'Baked Egg Carnivore Custard'

Serves 4

Ingredients

Milk 450ml – you can use goat, cow or sheep's milk

3 medium eggs, lightly beaten

1 – 3 teaspoons honey, optional

Double or single cream (you can use cream to replace up to 225ml of the milk for higher fat)

1 rasher of crispy crumbled bacon (for the topping)

Directions

<u>*For the topping:*</u>

If you are comfortable with the topping, simply prepare some bacon ahead of time. It should be desirably crispy but not burnt- such that it's easy to crumble.

Preheat your oven to 350 degrees F.

Add the eggs to a bowl and beat them lightly. Add the milk to the pan and heat it. If you want, you can add honey and cream until it's almost boiling. Pour the mixture over the beaten egg as you stir continuously.

Strain the mixture through a sieve into a 600ml oven proof dish so that any kind of lumps making the finished dish smoother are removed.

Put in the oven and bake at 350 degrees F for about 20 minutes. When ready (at first, the top has started to set and the center is a bit wobbly), take it out of the oven. Adjust the oven's temperature- if it has begun burning, you can turn the temperature down to 120 degrees C.

When the top is firm, sprinkle the crumbled bacon on top and put it back into the oven. Bake it for 20-40 more minutes until it's cooked through.

Take it out of the oven and let it cool.

Sausage Breakfast Sandwich

Serves 3

Ingredients

6 large eggs

Pinch red pepper flakes

Black pepper, freshly ground

3 slices cheddar

2 tablespoons heavy cream

Kosher salt

1 tablespoons butter

6 frozen sausage patties that have been heated according to package instructions

Directions

Add the eggs, heavy cream and red pepper flakes to a small bowl and whisk to combine.

Season the mixture generously with pepper and salt.

Set a non-stick skillet over medium heat and melt the butter.

Add roughly 1/3 of the eggs to the skillet and then lay a slice of cheese at the center to cover the cheese. Remove from the pan and repeat the process with the rest of the eggs.

The Carnivore Diet

Serve the eggs with the sausage patties and enjoy!

Ham & Cheese Egg Cups

Yields 12 cups

Ingredients

Cooking spray, for pan

1 cup shredded cheddar

Kosher salt

Chopped fresh parsley, for garnish

12 slices ham

12 large eggs

Freshly ground black pepper

Directions

Preheat your oven to 400 degrees.

Meanwhile, grease a 12-cup muffin tin lightly with cooking spray.

Line each cup with one slice of ham and then proceed to sprinkle with cheddar.

Next, crack an egg into every ham cup before seasoning with pepper and salt.

The Carnivore Diet

Bake the eggs until they're cooked through, for between 12 and 15 minutes, of course depending on how runny you want your yolks to be.

Garnish with parsley.

Serve and enjoy!

Butter Coffee

Serves 1

Ingredients

1 cup hot coffee freshly brewed

1 tablespoon MCT oil or coconut oil

2 tablespoons unsalted butter

Directions

Add all the ingredients to a blender and blend thoroughly until frothy and smooth.

Serve immediately and enjoy!

No-Bread Keto Breakfast Sandwich

Serves 2

Ingredients

2 tablespoons butter

Salt and pepper

2 ounces cheddar cheese or provolone cheese or Edam cheese, cut in thick slices

4 eggs

1 ounce smoked deli ham

A few drops of Tabasco or Worcestershire sauce (optional)

Directions

Add the butter to a frying pan set over medium heat.

Crack in the eggs and fry them well on both sides. Add some pepper and salt to taste.

For the base of each "sandwich," you're going to use a fried egg.

Put the pastrami/ cold cuts/ ham on each stack next and then add the cheese.

Then proceed to top each stack off with a fried egg. Leave it in the pan set over low heat, if you'd like the cheese to melt.

Sprinkle with Worcestershire sauce or Tabasco if you want, serve and enjoy immediately!

Ham And Swiss Omelet

Serves 1

Ingredients

1 tablespoon butter

3 tablespoons water

1/8 teaspoon pepper

1/4 cup shredded Swiss cheese

3 eggs

1/8 teaspoon salt

1/2 cup cubed fully cooked ham

Directions

Melt the butter over medium high heat in a small nonstick skillet and whisk the eggs, pepper, salt and water. Add the egg mixture to the skillet (the mixture should set at the edges immediately).

As the eggs are setting, go ahead and push the cooked edges towards the middle, allowing the uncooked sections to flow beneath.

When the eggs are well set, put the ham on one side and sprinkle with some cheese.

The Carnivore Diet

Fold the other side over filling and slide the omelet onto one plate.

Enjoy!

Breakfast Pockets

Serves 8

Ingredients

8 ounces mozzarella cheese, shredded or cubed

2/3 cup almond flour

1 egg

1 teaspoon salt

2 ounces cream cheese

1/3 cup coconut flour

2 teaspoon baking powder

For the filling:

2 eggs scrambled

1/2 cup of shredded cheddar cheese or other cheese of your choice

4 ounces Canadian bacon or other cooked breakfast meat

Directions

Preheat your oven to 350 degrees.

Place the cream cheese and mozzarella cheese in a microwave-safe bowl. Microwave for a minute, stir, microwave again for 30 seconds and stir once more. All the cheese, at this point, should be completely melted.

Microwave for 30 more seconds- it should currently be looking like cheese fondue.

Add the melted cheese and the rest of the dough ingredients to a food processor and process until everything forms uniform dough.

Alternatively, you can mix by hand, but ensure you thoroughly knead the dough.

Now form the dough into 8 pieces and press each one of them into a circle (about 6 inches) on a piece of parchment paper on a baking sheet. This will assist wet your hands.

Now divide the filling between each circle of dough, fold the edges in and crimp carefully to seal. Put it back on the parchment with the seam side down.

Bake for 20 – 25 minutes, until it turns golden brown.

Note:

These pockets are freezable. Cool them completely, put them in a plastic bag and freeze. Reheat for about 1 ½ minutes in the microwave. As usual, the microwave durations will vary a bit.

Lunch Recipes

The Best Garlic Cilantro Salmon

Serves 4

Ingredients

1 large salmon filet

4 cloves of garlic, minced

Kosher salt to taste

1 tablespoon butter (optional)

1 lemon

1/4 cup fresh cilantro leaves, roughly chopped

Freshly cracked black pepper to taste

Directions

Preheat your grill to 400 degrees F. Put the fish on a baking sheet lined with a baking sheet with the skin side facing down (this actually makes the cleanup easier). Avoid greasing the foil.

Squeeze your lemon over the salmon fillet.

Sprinkle the cilantro and garlic on top evenly.

Sprinkle with pepper and salt and if using, slice the butter and put the pieces over the top over the salmon evenly.

Place the foil with the fish on the preheated grill, or bake it in the preheated oven for about 7 minutes, depending on how thick it is.

Note: If you're grilling, skip the next step and keep grilling for roughly 15 minutes.

Turn it over to broil and keep cooking for 5-7 more minutes, until the top becomes nice and crispy.

Take the salmon out of the grill or oven and slide a flat spatula in between the fish and the skin. The skin should stick to the foil, making it easy to separate the fish from the skin. Serve immediately and enjoy.

Skillet Rib Eye Steaks

Serves 2

Ingredients

1 (1 1/4 pound) bone-in rib eye steak

2 teaspoons of chopped fresh rosemary leaves

1 tablespoon olive oil

1 teaspoon Stone House Seasoning

1 tablespoon unsalted butter

Directions

Put your rib eye on a sheet pan and rub the two sides with seasoning to coat. Make sure you press the seasoning to the meat. Sprinkle the dish with fresh rosemary leaves.

Refrigerate the steaks, covered, for up to three days.

When you're ready to cook your steaks, remove from the fridge and give it about 30 minutes to rest at room temperature.

To cook, set a medium skillet over medium heat.

Add olive oil and butter to the skillet and let the butter to melt completely.

Tilt the skillet from side to side so that the skillet is coated properly with the olive oil and butter.

Immerse the rib eye steak into the olive oil and butter and cook until the lower part of the steak browns and become caramelized, for about 5 minutes.

Turn the steak over and cook, while basting the steak constantly with the oil drippings and butter from the skillet, until this side of the steak turns brown and caramelized as well, for another five minutes, or to any temperature you desire for doneness.

Remove the steak out of the heat and let it rest on a carving board for about 5 minutes more.

Slice the steak using a sharp knife against the grain, making sure you don't remove the bone. Serve the stake slices on two plates and enjoy!

Note:

You can increase the number of steaks based on the total servings required.

Secondly, you should use an internal temp probe to check for your desired level of doneness. Medium well is between 150 and 160 degrees F, medium is between 140 and 150 degrees F, medium rare is between 130 and 140 degrees F and rare is between 120 degrees and 130 degrees F.

Olive Oil-Basted Grass-Fed Strip Steak

Serves 4

Ingredients

3 tablespoons olive oil, divided

1 teaspoon kosher salt, divided

1 (3-inch) rosemary sprig

Rosemary leaves (optional)

2 (8-ounce) grass-fed New York strip steaks, trimmed

1 teaspoon freshly ground black pepper, divided

1 garlic clove, crushed

Directions

Set your grill pan over medium high heat. Brush one tablespoon of oil on steaks, and sprinkle each one of them with ½ teaspoon of pepper and salt.

Add the garlic, sprig of rosemary and one tablespoon of oil to the pan and then add the steaks.

Cook them for 9 minutes, until the steaks reach the desired level of doneness; turn them and baste them with oil once every minute.

The Carnivore Diet

Put the steaks on a chopping board, and leave them to set for five minutes. Slice the steaks across the grain and put them on a platter. Sprinkle them with the rest of the pepper and salt, and if you want, garnish with rosemary leaves.

Vivica's Keto Roast Chicken

Serves 8

Ingredients

1 whole organic chicken

2 garlic cloves

1 teaspoon herbes de provence

2 sprigs organic rosemary

1 tablespoon coarse sea salt

Directions

Have the chicken set to room temperature.

Preheat your oven to 350 degrees. Meanwhile, remove the chicken from the packaging, and rinse under cold water properly. Put it on a glass pyrex or a baking pan with the breast facing up.

Stuff the cavity using the garlic cloves and rosemary; you don't have to peel them.

Sprinkle half of the Herbes de Provence and salt on the breast. Turn the chicken breast side down, and sprinkle with the rest of the herb and salt mix over the top.

Bake the chicken for roughly 1 ½ hours at 350 degrees. The skin should be nice and brown when the chicken is ready.

You need to however note that the cooking time might change a bit depending on your oven temperature, as well as the cooking time.

You can check for doneness by pulling the leg apart from the body, or cutting the area between the leg and body. The meat should be pink and any juice coming from inside should be clear.

Serve the dish with a desired side dish and enjoy!

Grilled Split Lobster

Serves 2

Ingredients

2 tablespoons vegetable oil, plus more for grill

Kosher salt and freshly ground black pepper

2 (1½-pound) live lobsters

Melted unsalted butter, hot sauce, and lemon wedges (to serve)

Directions

Set your grill to medium high heat and oil the grate. Put the lobsters in a freezer to chill for 15 minutes- so that their nervous system slows down to have an easy time doing the rest.

Transfer one of them to a chopping board, with the belly side facing down, and the head facing you. Hold the tail using a kitchen towel (the lobster should be quite inactive now) and bisect the body and head lengthwise in one swoop. Turn the lobster around and cut it lengthwise through the tail. Remove any eggs or tomalley and reserve them if you want.

Now rub the lobster's cut side with two tablespoons of oil and season with pepper and salt. Grill the cut side down, while pressing the claws against the grill, until the meat is almost cooked through, for 6-8 minutes. Turn them and grill until the shells are charred a bit and the meat is almost cooked through, for between 6 and 8 minutes (the meat in the tail should be firm and opaque).

Remove the lobsters from the grill and serve it with hot sauce, butter, and squeeze over some lemon wedges.

Enjoy!

Grilled Shrimp Seasoning

Serves 4

Ingredients

The shrimp seasoning:

1 teaspoon garlic powder

1 teaspoon Italian seasoning

1 teaspoon kosher salt

1/4 - 1/2 teaspoon cayenne pepper — you can use 1/4 if you're sensitive to spice

The grilling:

2 tablespoons extra virgin olive oil

Canola or vegetable oil for the grill

Juice of ½ small lemon (about 1 tablespoon)

1 pound of peeled and deveined shrimp

Directions

Preheat your outdoor or indoor grill to high heat. Preheat the broiler to cook the shrimp using the oven. If you're going to broil, line a sheet pan with a foil and coat with some non-stick spray.

Add the cayenne, Italian seasoning, salt and garlic powder to a large mixing bowl and stir them together. Drizzle in the lemon juice and olive oil, and stir everything together into a paste.

Add the shrimp and toss thoroughly to coat. If you're using a smaller shrimp, thread them on clean metal or wooden skewers previously soaked in water for not less than one hour.

Brush the grill pan or the regular grill using the canola oil. Broil or grill the shrimp for 2-3 minutes on each side, until pink and opaque. You can turn it once half way through, and perhaps throw away the additional spices or liquid that's left at the bottom of the bowl.

Serve immediately and enjoy!

Note:

You will enjoy grilled shrimp the most when you eat it the day you make it. You can however store it for up to two days.

Duck Leg Confit

Serves 4

Ingredients

4 duck leg portions with their thighs attached (make sure to trim and reserve the excess fat)

4 cups of duck fat or olive oil

1/2 teaspoon freshly ground black pepper

4 bay leaves

1 1/2 teaspoons black peppercorns

10 garlic cloves

4 sprigs fresh thyme

1/2 teaspoon table salt

1 tablespoon of kosher salt (plus 1/8 teaspoon)

Directions

Put the legs on a platter, with the skin side facing down. Sprinkle with one tablespoon of the black pepper and kosher salt and put the bay leaves, sprigs of thyme and garlic cloves on each one of the two leg portions.

Put the rest of the 2 leg portions on top, flesh to flesh. Put the reserved fat from the ducks in the bottom of a plastic container or glass and top with the now sandwiched leg portions.

Sprinkle with the rest of the kosher salt, cover, and put in the fridge to chill for about 12 hours.

Preheat your oven to 300 degrees F.

Get the duck out of the refrigerator. Remove the bay leaves, duck fat, thyme and garlic and reserve. Rinse the duck in cool water, making sure to rub off a bit of the pepper and salt properly. Pat dry with paper towels.

Add the reserved duck fat, garlic, thyme and bay leaves in the bottom of an enameled cast-iron pot, and sprinkle evenly with salt and peppercorns.

Lay the duck on top, with the skin side facing down, and add the duck fat or olive oil. Bake, covered for 2 ½ - 3 hours or until the meat pulls away from the bone.

Now get the duck out of the fat, strain the fat and set aside.

Sear the duck legs skin side down in a hot pan for 3 to 4 minutes, until the skin is crispy and golden, or if you want to save for later, pick the meat carefully from the bones and store it in a stoneware container.

Using a bit of the strained fat, cover the meat to make a layer- about ¼ inch thick.

You can store the duck confit in the fridge for up to a month

Beef (Heart) Steak

Serves 2

Ingredients

1 tablespoon ghee

2 tablespoons of olive oil (you can use plain or rosemary infused)

4 slices of beef heart 1-inch thick

Salt and pepper for seasoning

Directions

Get the heart slices from the marinade and pat them dry.

Then set a cast iron skillet on a high flame and allow it to heat up for 2/3 minutes.

Lay the meat on the skillet; you should ensure the temperature is high enough to sizzle.

Prepare each slice for five minutes per side, until the outside is nicely browned on the outside but still pink in the middle.

Drizzle the slices with the rosemary-infused olive oil.

Serve and enjoy!

<u>*Note:*</u>

The Carnivore Diet

To remove the strong blood odor, marinate the heart into apple cider vinegar about 24 hours before you start cooking.

Grilled Beef Liver

Serves 5

Ingredients

1 pound beef liver cut into thin slices

1 clove garlic, crushed

1 teaspoon salt

½ cup olive oil

1 tablespoon fresh mint, finely chopped

¼ teaspoon black pepper, freshly ground

Direction

Set your grill pan over medium-high heat and preheat it.

Rinse the liver under cold running water thoroughly, making sure to wash out all the traces of blood.

Pat it dry using a kitchen paper.

Grab a sharp knife and remove all the tough veins, if there're any, and cut into thin slices crosswise.

Add the pepper, salt, mint, crushed garlic and olive oil to a small bowl and mix until well integrated.

Brush the liver slices with this mixture generously and grill on each side for 5-7 minutes.

Serve and enjoy!

Moroccan Liver Kebabs

Serves 4

Ingredients

4 ounces of kidney fat (suet)

1.1 pounds of calf or lamb liver less than 2 days old (young liver is better)

<u>The marinade:</u>

1 teaspoon salt

1 tablespoon ground sweet paprika

1/2 tsp ground cumin

<u>Condiments:</u>

1 teaspoon cayenne pepper, optional

1 teaspoon salt

1 teaspoon ground cumin

Directions

<u>For the preparation of the liver:</u>

Cut out the transparent membrane that surrounds the liver and cut the liver into 2 cm thick cubes.

Cut the suet/fat into tiny cubes as well and mix them with the liver cubes; add the spices. Cover and leave for not more than one hour to marinate (it can also take as long as overnight) in your refrigerator.

For the grilling:

Set up your grill and light the charcoal. When the flames go out, the coals develop a thin grey cover; consider the grill ready for cooking.

As the grill heats up, thread the liver cubes on the skewer, carefully alternating a few pieces with a kidney fat cube; avoid leaving any space between the pieces or over packing the skewers. As a rule of thumb, you can have between 6 and 8 cubes of liver per skewer.

Now start grilling the kebabs, making sure to turn to cook on all sides, until the liver cooks through and is seared a bit, but still a little spongy when you squeeze it.

Serve immediately and enjoy.

You should serve hot from the grill; have the meat sprinkled with cayenne powder and cumin or have the spices as condiments on the side.

Lastly, ensure you have some hot Moroccan tea to go with it to get the most of this dish.

Note:

I would advise you try and choose fresh liver – it should not be older than 2 days old, and should have the least veins and ventricles possible. Calf liver is generally more preferable to lamb liver because of its texture, and also because it is very easy to handle.

Secondly, you have two options when it comes to going about this recipe. You can cube and marinate the liver as I have described above, or you can slice the liver into steaks about 2 cm thick and pre-grill them for one minute on all sides to sear the liver before you cube and marinate.

Lastly, you can follow this recipe to make Moroccan kidney and heart kebabs/ skewers.

Fresh Oysters

Serves 2

Ingredients

6 oysters, from sustainable sources

Tabasco sauce, optional

1-2 lemons, optional

Directions

When you purchase your oysters, ensure they are well closed and are heavy in the hand. The oysters should ideally be straight from the sea when you cook them.

So rinse them gently in cold water before you begin their preparation; this can be a bit tricky so you need to be very careful. Grab an oyster knife that is a bit blunt, and also thick and short. Avoid using an ordinary kitchen knife because it's very easy for it to snap at the tip, making it dangerous to use. If you don't have an oyster knife, use a good screw driver to open them up.

Now hold the oyster on a cutting board with the curved side facing down using a folded kitchen cloth (well placed in between your hand and the shell). This will enable you to have a good grip and shield your hand.

Now look at the hinge between the top and bottom shells, and poke the tip of the knife into the crack. Push a bit hard and work it in there; you should be able to open the top shell off. Since this is not a very easy task, you might want to try to get a hang of it before dinner by trying a couple of times. You may also consider wearing an apron just in case you get dirty.

When you finally open the oyster, discard the top shell and if there's any seawater in the oyster's bottom shell, do keep it in there.

Pick out any shell fragments and put the oyster on a plate with some crushed ice and a mound of rock salt at the center.

Season it in any way you like- Tabasco or lemon juice is a good idea. Enjoy the lovely fresh oyster.

Grilled Lamb Chops

Yields 8 chops

Ingredients

8 1 1/4 inches thick lamb chops

2 tablespoons of chopped fresh rosemary (don't use dried rosemary)

1 teaspoon kosher salt

3 tablespoons olive oil

3 cloves garlic minced

Freshly ground black pepper to taste

Directions

Set your stove top grill pan to medium heat and preheat it.

Arrange the lamb chops on a plate in one layer.

Add the marinade ingredients to a small bowl and combine them. Spoon this mixture over both sides of the lamb chops evenly.

Grill the chops at 135 degrees F for medium rare- for between 3 and 4 minutes on each side to achieve your preferred level of doneness.

Next, transfer the chops to a platter and allow them to rest for ten minutes before you serve.

Note:

This recipe is for lamb rib chops but will work just fine with loin chops (lamb)- all you need is to increase the time of cooking by 2-3 minutes per side.

If you want to cook them on the stove top, preheat your grill pan over medium high heat and cook as you would using the grill.

AIP Bacon-Wrapped Salmon

Serves 1

Ingredients

2 filets of salmon, fresh or frozen

1 tablespoon of olive oil

Lemon wedges, to serve

4 slices of bacon

2 tablespoons of tarragon, to garnish

Directions

Preheat your oven to 350 degrees F. Meanwhile, pat the salmon fillets dry and wrap the bacon around them.

Put the fillets on a roasting tray, drizzle with olive oil and bake for about 15- 20 minutes.

Garnish the dish with lemon wedges and chopped tarragon.

Serve and enjoy!

Dinner Recipes

Baked Chicken Breast

Ingredients

1 chicken breast

1 tablespoon ghee (you can also use olive or coconut oil)

1 teaspoon sea salt

1 teaspoon garlic powder

2 cloves garlic, chopped (you can use 2 teaspoons of garlic powder)

1 teaspoon chives, diced (optional)

Directions

Preheat your oven to 180 degrees C.

Put the chicken breast on a small aluminum foil and then add the chopped fresh garlic, garlic powder, ghee and salt over it.

Now rub everything gently over the chicken breast and fold up the foil such that the entire chicken breast is fully covered.

Put the chicken on a baking tray, put the tray in the oven and bake for 30 minutes. When you insert a thermometer in the middle of the chicken when the time elapses, it should read above 75 degrees C; it should also be well cooked through-without any pink at the center.

Cut the chicken in half or into any desired number of slices; sprinkle the diced chives over it. Serve and enjoy with more salt to taste, and ghee.

Pressure Cooked Pork Loin Roast

Serves 9

Ingredients

3 pounds pork loin roast

1 teaspoon dried oregano

1 teaspoon ground cumin

1 teaspoon coriander

1 tablespoon oil

2 cups chicken bone broth

1 teaspoon onion powder

1 teaspoon garlic powder

1 teaspoon dried thyme

1/2 teaspoon kosher salt or more if desired

2 cloves garlic minced

Directions

Add the salt, coriander, thyme, cumin, garlic powder, oregano and onion powder to a small bowl and combine. Rub the seasoning mix into the pork loin roast.

Add the oil to a pressure cooker, heat it up; sauté and stir fry the garlic until fragrant. Add the pork loin and cook until all sides are browned.

Get the roast out of the pot and deglaze it with half of the bone broth.

Add the rest of the broth and put the rack in the bottom of the pot.

Place the pork loin on top of the rack and pressure cook on high. After about 25 minutes, perform a quick pressure release. Get the roast out of the pot and let it sit for 10 – 15 minutes before you go ahead and start slicing.

Enjoy!

Crispy Oven Roasted Salmon

Serves 3

Ingredients

1 pound salmon fillet

1/4 teaspoon sea salt

1 tablespoon coconut oil

1/2 teaspoon mixed herbs of choice (thyme, marjoram, oregano etc.)

Directions

Line your baking sheet with parchment paper. Grease it with coconut oil and preheat your oven to 425 degrees F.

Put the salmon fillet on the baking sheet, with the skin side facing down, and season lightly with herbs of choice and salt, to taste.

Pour one tablespoon of coconut oil over the salmon and cook until the level of crispiness you want is attained, which should take about 20 minutes.

Serve the dish immediately and enjoy!

Put it in a glass container and store it in your fridge for up to two days.

Pinchos De Pollo

Serves 4

Ingredients

1 tablespoon minced garlic

½ teaspoon of freshly ground black pepper

1 tablespoon extra-virgin olive oil

1½ pound boneless, skinless chicken breast

½ teaspoon fine Himalayan salt

2 teaspoons minced fresh oregano or 1 teaspoon dried

1 tablespoon of lime juice, freshly squeezed

Directions

Get 7 to 9 skewers ready, and if you're going to use bamboo or wooden skewers, start by soaking them in water for at least 30 minutes before you can start grilling.

Add oil, lime juice, oregano, pepper, salt, and the garlic to a bowl and stir carefully to form a paste.

Then cut the chicken breasts into 2.5 cm thick chunks and put them in a glass container that has a lid.

Pour the marinade over the chicken and stir thoroughly to combine.

Cover the chicken well and refrigerate for not less than 2 hours or even overnight if you wish.

Now prepare your grill for medium heat (between 325 and 375 degrees F) for direct cooking. This may take between 15 and 20 minutes depending on the kind of grill you're using.

Now remove the chicken from the fridge and thread it onto the skewers, making sure to spread each piece as flat as you can; leave a tiny space between each piece though.

When the grill heats up, brush the cooking grates clean, if you want- so that you don't have a problem with sticking.

Next, over direct medium heat, grill the kebabs, making sure to keep the lid closed as much as you can, until the chicken is no longer pink and feels firm to touch, about 8 and 10 minutes. Make sure to turn once or twice in course of the cooking. Try to avoid overcooking.

Remove the chicken from the grill and serve immediately.

Enjoy!

Whole Roasted Beef Tenderloin

Serves 10

Ingredients

1 raw, trimmed whole beef tenderloin (without tail) – about 4 pounds

1 tablespoon olive oil

1/4 teaspoon ground black pepper

4 ounces deli sliced prosciutto

1 tablespoon raw garlic, finely chopped or crushed

1 tablespoon kosher salt

1 tablespoon fresh parsley, chopped

Directions

Preheat your oven to 425 degrees F.

Meanwhile, add the fresh parsley, pepper, salt, olive oil and garlic to a small bowl and mix to combine. Place your tenderloin on a chopping board.

Rub the garlic mixture all over and press it into the tenderloin on all sides. Wrap the tenderloin in overlapping prosciutto ribbons gently until well covered.

Put the tenderloin in a roasting pan or a cookie sheet, and roast it for 26 -28 minutes at 425 degrees F for rare. Otherwise, roast it for 30 minutes (for medium rare) 35 - 40 minutes for "well done". Don't forget that these are just general guidelines; ovens can vary, just as the tenderloin thicknesses do. So it's prudent to make sure you use a meat thermometer to make sure it's done the way you like.

Take it out of the oven and give it about 10 minutes to rest before you start slicing.

Serve warm or cold and enjoy!

Coconut-Lime Skirt Steak

Serves 4

Ingredients

1/2 cup coconut oil, melted

Zest of one lime

1 teaspoon grated fresh ginger

3/4 teaspoon sea salt

2 tablespoons freshly squeezed lime juice from one lime

1 tablespoons minced garlic

1 teaspoon red pepper flakes (depending on how spicy you like it)

2 pounds grass-fed skirt steak (you can cut it into sections)

Directions

Add the lime juice, coconut oil, ginger, red pepper flakes, ginger, garlic, salt and zest to a large bowl and mix well.

Add the steaks and rub or toss with the marinade. When you're done, the coconut oil will harden and that's fine. Allow the meat to marinate for 20 or so minutes, at room temperature.

Now set a large skillet over medium-high heat and transfer the steak to it. If it doesn't fit, cut in half against the grain. If you find that some of the marinade is still stuck to the bowl, just spoon it out into the pan so that it cooks with the steak.

Now sear the steak on the two sides until it cooks to the level of doneness you desire, for between 4 and 5 minutes per side. Skirt steak generally cooks fast.

Slice, serve and enjoy!

Philly Cheese Steak Casserole

Servings 6

Ingredients

1 1/2 pounds lean ground beef

1/2 yellow onion

1 teaspoon seasoned salt

4 large eggs

1 teaspoon hot sauce

2 bell peppers

1 clove garlic

4 slices Provolone cheese

1/4 cup heavy cream

1 teaspoon Worcestershire sauce

Directions

Preheat your oven to 350 degrees, and then spray your 9 x 9 baking dish with non-stick spray.

Dice the onions and peppers into tiny pieces, and mince the garlic.

Add the ground beef to the skillet and cook over medium heat, crumbling often as it cooks.

When the beef breaks apart, but is still pink, add the onion, garlic, peppers and seasoned salt. Keep cooking while stirring often until the beef cooks through and the condiments have softened slightly.

Drain the grease and add the mixture to the prepared baking dish. Cut the cheese into bite-size pieces and scatter them over the beef mixture.

Whisk the eggs, hot sauce, cream and Worcestershire sauce in your mixing bowl until well integrated.

Pour the egg mixture over the beef and put the dish in the oven; bake until the eggs set, for about 35 minutes.

Allow the dish to sit for five minutes before slicing and serving.

Mini Cheeseburger Meatloaves

Serves 4

Ingredients

1 1/2 pounds ground beef

12 bacon slices

1 egg

1/4 cup homemade ketchup

Fresh parsley to garnish

1 minced onion

2 minced garlic cloves

1/2 cup aged cheddar cheese, cubed (optional)

1/2 tablespoon of dried oregano

Sea salt and freshly ground black pepper

Directions

Preheat your oven to 400 degrees F.

Mix the onion, garlic, egg, oregano, ketchup and cheese with the ground beef until everything is well combined.

Grab a muffin pan and add one slice of bacon beside and around each hole. Fill each hole surrounded with the bacon with the beef mixture, and shape it into little muffins.

Put it in the oven and bake for between 30 and 35 minutes.

Allow to cool before you remove from the pan, for about five minutes. Serve with fresh parsley and enjoy!

Grilled Marinated Venison Steak

Serves 1

Ingredients

8 ounces venison steak

Marinade

1/2 can of frozen concentrate apple juice (6 ounces)

1/4 teaspoon ground garlic powder

1/4 teaspoon ground black pepper

1/2 teaspoon ground cinnamon

1/4 teaspoon ground onion powder

Directions

Add the marinade ingredients to a microwave safe bowl and mix them together until well integrated.

Put the bowl in the microwave and then cook on high for about 15 seconds so that the cinnamon dissolves.

Place the steak in a sealable container and pour the marinade nicely over it.

Marinate for 8 hours or more. Now grill the steak over a medium hot grill for a short while (since venison cooks fast).

Note:

The Carnivore Diet

To grill the venison, simply sear your steak on one side, and then flip it, and cook the steak without flipping it again. Remember that venison is very lean, so it will only take between 3 and 5 minutes to be ready- of course, depending on how hot your grill is. Just try to avoid overcooking it. It should have a nice pink color in the middle.

Enjoy!

Crockpot Venison BBQ

Serves 3

Ingredients

1 pound venison stew meat

1/3 cup barbecue sauce

1 tablespoon onion powder

1/3 cup water

1 tablespoon garlic salt

Directions

Marinate the venison in garlic salt, onion powder and barbecue sauce.

Switch on the slow cooker and set to low, add water and then add the venison mixture and combine until level.

Top this with a little more barbecue sauce if you want and cook for 4-6 minutes on low heat.

When ready, transfer the meat to a cutting board and chop it.

Add the meat back to the sauce when you're done.

Enjoy!

Smoked Duck or Goose

Serves 1

Ingredients

1 small wild goose or wild duck

1/4 cup of thick maple syrup

Salt

Directions

Salt the duck properly within the cavity, and then paint the outer flesh using the maple syrup. Salt this outer area as well.

Place a drip pan underneath a smoker and set the bird in the smoker.

Smoke over apple wood, about 200 - 225 degrees, for four hours.

Each hour, baste the ducks with the maple syrup and then allow to cool completely when fully smoked before carving.

Either serve as a cold cut or at room temperature. You can carve the breast whole and sear in a pan.

Slice and enjoy with anything you want.

Keto Pizza

Serves 5

Ingredients

24 ounces of shredded cheese (I recommend mozzarella)

8 ounces ground pork (you could also use what is known as the "breakfast sausage")

A bit of butter

Cooking sheet

1 pound of ground beef

A package of pepperoni

Parchment paper

Directions

Begin by preheating your oven to 425 degrees.

Melt the butter in a pan and sauté the one pound of ground beef and the pork.

Now get a parchment paper and lay it nicely on your cooking sheet. Now spread out 16 ounces of cheese on it evenly.

Next, strain the meat and spread it over the cheese evenly.

Sprinkle some extra cheese on it and then layer the pepperoni.

The Carnivore Diet

Now put it in the oven and let it cook for roughly 16 minutes. After it cools for a short while, the cheese will become stiff and will hold up like any regular slice of pizza.

Serve and enjoy!

Snack/Appetizer/Dessert Recipes

Honey Sriracha Lime Duck Legs

Serves 6

Ingredients

3 pounds of duck legs

3/4 cup sriracha hot sauce

3 tablespoons honey, or to taste

Salt

Juice of 2 limes

1 tablespoon soy sauce

Directions

Salt the duck legs properly and arrange them in one layer, skin down, in a sheet pan or roasting pan.

Put them in the oven and set it to 400 degrees F. Avoid preheating the oven since you should look to have the temperature come up gradually so that a bit of the duck's fat renders and moistens the pan; this ensures the legs don't stick to it.

Roast for about 90 minutes- 2 hours, or until tender. After this time, you might have a couple of legs that are still tough but since you're working with wild food, you should expect it.

Now if you're working with domesticated legs, you might only require roughly one hour. You however need to note that in the oven used to prepare this recipe, it takes half an hour to get to 400 degrees F, so if your oven heats up quickly, you can begin at 350 degrees F for half an hour before then jacking up the heat. Secondly, you need to note that pre-braised legs only require between 20 and 30 minutes to crisp up.

In the meantime, combine the rest of the ingredients together in a little pot and warm just enough to include the honey.

When the legs are tender, remove them from the oven but keep it on. Add them to a large bowl gently so that the meat doesn't come off the bone, and add the sauce nicely over them.

Toss them gently to combine and take them back to the baking sheet, skin side facing up, and then put them back in the oven. Don't take your eyes off the wings; when you begin seeing some char on the sauce, which will caramelize pretty fast, pull them out.

Serve with the rest of the sauce in the mixing bowl and enjoy!

Elk Burgers

Serves 4

Ingredients

1 pound elk meat

1 teaspoon minced garlic

1 tablespoon red wine vinegar

1/2 large red onion chopped small, diced

Ground black pepper

1 tablespoon Worcestershire sauce

1/2 packages container blue cheese

Dash paprika

Red pepper flakes

Dash salt

Directions

Combine the ingredients together and form patties, making between 4 and 6.

Cook over medium-high or medium heat and flip every 5 or so minutes.

Serve and enjoy with anything nice!

Papa's Duck Poppers

Serves 4

Ingredients

4 wild duck breast halves, bones removed

1 jar of jalapeno pepper slices

1 box of wooden toothpicks

1 bottle of Italian Dressing

1 regular brick of cream cheese (cool to make it sliceable)

1 package of uncooked bacon (thick cut)

Directions

If the duck breasts are clean, de-bone them and remove the skin. Put the breasts in a container or a zip-lock bag and pour some Italian dressing over them nicely.

Marinate the breasts in the fridge for 3-6 hours.

Preheat the grill. In the meantime, remove the breasts from the marinade and butterfly them well such that there is a cavity at the center.

Add a slice of cream cheese and some jalapeno peppers into the breast cavity.

Fold the breast back over in such a way that it surrounds the peppers and cream cheese. Now wrap the breast with the bacon, and secure them from opening with the toothpicks.

When the grill is set, grill the breasts for about 5 minutes per side- medium rare is ideal here.

Remove them from the grill and serve the breasts as entrees or cut them into tiny pieces and eat them as appetizers.

<u>Note:</u>

Soak the breasts using salted ice water for about 30 minutes before you add to the Italian dressing so that some of the wild game taste and blood is removed. Rinse well and pat dry before you add to the dressing.

Enjoy!

Ham Pizza Snacks

Serves 10

Ingredients

7 1/2 ounces refrigerated biscuit dough

1/4 cup pizza sauce

2/3 cup mozzarella cheese (shredded)

Nonstick cooking spray

2/3 cup ham (diced)

Directions

Spray your cookie sheet with nonstick spray.

Separate the biscuits and flatten them on the cookie sheet, making sure to leave space between so that the edges don't touch.

Spread the pizza sauce on the biscuits and top each one of them with one tablespoon of diced ham, and another tablespoon of shredded cheese.

Put in the oven and bake at 400 degrees F for 8 -10 minutes. The biscuits should be light brown and the cheese in molten form.

Pizza Cup Snacks

Serves 4

Ingredients

1 can refrigerated biscuits (12 ounces -10 biscuits)

1 jar (14 ounce) pizza sauce

1/2 pound ground beef

1/2 cup shredded mozzarella cheese (about 2 ounces)

Directions

Preheat your oven to 375 degrees F. Press each biscuit in the sides and bottom of each cup in a 12-cup muffin pan. Chill them until they're all set to fill.

Add the ground beef to a 10-inch skillet set over medium-high heat, drain and stir in the sauce and heat through.

Spoon the beef mixture into the prepared muffin cups evenly, and bake for 15 minutes.

Next, sprinkle the beef mixture with cheese and bake for 5 more minutes or until the cheese melts and the biscuits are golden.

Let it stand for five minutes before you serve.

Remove the pizza cups from the muffin pan gently and serve.

Tangy Barbecue Wings

Ingredients

5 pounds chicken wings

2/3 cup white vinegar

1/2 cup molasses

1 teaspoon salt

1/2 teaspoon chili powder

2 1/2 cups ketchup

2/3 cup honey

2 to 3 tablespoons hot pepper sauce

1 teaspoon Worcestershire sauce

1/2 teaspoon onion powder

1/2 to 1 teaspoon liquid smoke, optional

Directions

Preheat your oven to 375 degrees F.

Cut through the two wing joints using a sharp knife and throw away the wing tips.

Arrange the rest of the wing pieces in two greased baking pans (15 x 10 x 1 inches). Bake for half an hour, drain, turn the wings and then bake for 20 -25 more minutes or until the juices run clear.

In the meantime, combine the rest of the ingredients in a large saucepan and bring to a boil.

Reduce the heat and simmer for half an hour, uncovered, and stirring occasionally.

Drain the wings and put one third of the chicken in a slow cooker.

Top it with one third of the sauce, and repeat layers twice.

Cover well and cook for 3-4 hours on low. Stir properly before you serve.

Enjoy!

Note:

You can substitute wingettes or uncooked wing sections for whole chicken wings.

Pork Satay

Serves 20

Ingredients

1 pound pork tenderloin, cut into 1/4-inch slices

1/3 cup reduced-sodium soy sauce

3 tablespoons brown sugar

3 tablespoons Thai chili sauce

2 teaspoons minced garlic

1/3 cup creamy peanut butter

2 teaspoons lime juice

2 green onions, sliced

3 tablespoons minced fresh cilantro

2 tablespoons sesame oil

3 tablespoons hot water

Directions

Add all the ingredients except the pork, peanut butter, hot water and lime juice to a small bowl and mix well.

Set aside ¼ cup for the dipping sauce. Add the rest of the sauce to a large re-sealable plastic bag and then add the pork. Seal the bag and turn to coat.

Refrigerate for half an hour.

Drain and throw away the marinade. Thread the slices of pork onto 20 soaked wooden skewers or metal skewers.

Put the skewers on a greased baking pan measuring 15 x 10 x 1 inches. Broil for 3-4 minutes on each side, or until you note the meat juices running clear.

To create the sauce, add the water and peanut butter to a small bowl and combine.

Add the lime juice and the reserved soy sauce mixture as you stir until smooth.

Serve with skewers and enjoy!

Tavuk Göğsü

Serves 6

Ingredients

1 chicken breast

1 1/4 cup heavy cream

3/4 cup sugar

3 1/2 cups milk

1/4 teaspoon salt

5 tablespoons rice flour

Directions

Put the chicken breast in your pan with some water and bring to a boil.

Reduce the heat and simmer until the meat cooks properly; drain it and tear the meat into fine threads.

Add a little milk to the rice flour to moisten it a bit, and then add the remaining milk to a sauce pan containing the sugar, salt and cream; bring to a boil.

Add some spoonfuls of the hot liquid to the rice flour and pour the entire mixture into the pan.

Take some time to beat it vigorously and keep cooking over low heat, stirring often so that it doesn't stick to the floor of the pan, until the mixture starts thickening. Beat in the fine threads of chicken and keep cooking the mixture until it becomes very thick.

At this point, you can either cook your pudding or eat it plain. Of course, you can garnish with anything you love if you want to.

As an alternative, you can tip it into a heavy-based pan and put it over the heat for between 5 -10 minutes so that the bottom of the pudding burns, and then move the pan around to have the pudding evenly burnt.

Leave it to cool while inside the pan before cutting it into rectangles. Simply lift out the rectangles using a spatula then roll them into logs.

Serve slightly cooled or at room temperature and enjoy!

Lattice Mincemeat Dessert Tart

Ingredients

1¼ pound home-made mincemeat

2½ ounces butter

A pinch salt

10 ounces plain flour

2½ ounces lard

The topping:

Icing sugar

A little milk

Directions

Sift the salt and flour into a mixing bowl to make the pastry. Then proceed to rub the fats into the mixture until everything looks like fine crumbs. Now add some cold water- just enough to make dough that leaves your bowl very clean. Put the dough inside a polythene bag and let it rest in the fridge for about 20 minutes before you roll out.

When ready, cut off 1/3 of the pastry and store it for later use. Roll out the rest of the pastry and use it to line a prepared tin. Spoon the minced meat over the pastry, making sure to spread it out evenly using a palette knife.

The Carnivore Diet

Grab a pastry brush and dampen the edges of the pastry with water- all round.

Roll out the rest of the pastry to an oblong strip that measures roughly 10 x 7 inches, and then cut the pastry by running a lattice cutter on its length. Make sure you firmly press as you go, and keep doing it in parallel over the oblong. Using both hands, ease out the lattice gently as a way to pull it open. Now when it's completely open, you'll have a square - about 10 inches- that you need to lift gently on to the pie.

Gently press the edges of the lattice against the pastry lining, and trim off the excess parts all round. Brush the lattice, this time using milk, and bake the tart on a baking sheet on the top most shelf of the oven for between 20 and 30 minutes. Dust the tart using icing sugar before you serve, and hand round the chilled butter separately.

Conclusion

I believe you now understand what the carnivore diet is all about. We've talked about the meaning of the diet, how it works and the benefits you stand to gain from it. We've also looked at the potential dangers of consuming a diet mainly composed of plants and all the recipes you need to get yourself started in the right direction.

As you've also seen, the carnivore diet meals are not as boring as most people think. There are many ways to prepare meat and animal products, some of which are evident in this book. You can be as creative as you want as well with your recipes as long as you ensure your diet is largely carnivore.

Before I leave, I have to reiterate the fact we've been eating meat for three million years. Its nutrient and caloric density rendered our large guts useless; they were no longer needed to digest fibrous plant matter and create huge, energy hogging brains. You'll never find one culture on earth that entirely abstained or abstains from animal product- because of its value. Almost every person on earth who lived ate meat when he or she was lucky to get it.

You know what to do from here, don't you?

Quoted Studies

I have arranged these in the order in which they have been mentioned throughout the book so you can flip back and forth for easy reading.

https://www.ncbi.nlm.nih.gov/pubmed/5046723

https://www.ncbi.nlm.nih.gov/pubmed/21239090

https://www.ncbi.nlm.nih.gov/pubmed/21239090

https://www.ncbi.nlm.nih.gov/pmc/articles/PMC2903695/

https://www.ncbi.nlm.nih.gov/pmc/articles/PMC5332116/

https://www.ncbi.nlm.nih.gov/pmc/articles/PMC5946249/

https://www.ncbi.nlm.nih.gov/pmc/articles/PMC3205262/

https://www.ncbi.nlm.nih.gov/pmc/articles/PMC5859338/

https://www.ncbi.nlm.nih.gov/books/NBK10807/

https://link.springer.com/article/10.1007%2FBF02253527

https://academic.oup.com/jn/article/130/4/915S/4686622

https://www.ncbi.nlm.nih.gov/pubmed/12481981

https://academic.oup.com/jn/article/130/4/915S/4686622

https://www.ncbi.nlm.nih.gov/pubmed/12481981

https://www.ncbi.nlm.nih.gov/pmc/articles/PMC3698427/

https://academic.oup.com/jn/article/130/4/915S/4686622

https://www.ncbi.nlm.nih.gov/pubmed/12481981

https://www.ncbi.nlm.nih.gov/pubmed/10736351

https://www.ncbi.nlm.nih.gov/pmc/articles/PMC5859338/

https://www.ncbi.nlm.nih.gov/pmc/articles/PMC5968124/

https://www.ncbi.nlm.nih.gov/pmc/articles/PMC4517012/

https://www.sciencedaily.com/releases/2013/08/130829092648.htm

https://www.ncbi.nlm.nih.gov/pubmed/26895672

https://www.ncbi.nlm.nih.gov/pubmed/20201035

https://www.ncbi.nlm.nih.gov/pmc/articles/PMC6327661/

https://www.ncbi.nlm.nih.gov/pmc/articles/PMC3899416/

https://www.ncbi.nlm.nih.gov/pmc/articles/PMC5452247/

https://www.ncbi.nlm.nih.gov/pmc/articles/PMC4532752/

https://www.ncbi.nlm.nih.gov/pmc/articles/PMC2716748/

https://www.ncbi.nlm.nih.gov/pubmed/16652223

https://www.ncbi.nlm.nih.gov/pmc/articles/PMC3826507/

https://www.ncbi.nlm.nih.gov/pmc/articles/PMC387257/

https://www.ncbi.nlm.nih.gov/pmc/articles/PMC5385025/

https://www.hindawi.com/journals/bmri/2016/5828959/

https://www.ncbi.nlm.nih.gov/pmc/articles/PMC4369670/

https://www.ncbi.nlm.nih.gov/pmc/articles/PMC3249386/

https://www.ncbi.nlm.nih.gov/pubmed/27285936

https://www.ncbi.nlm.nih.gov/pubmed/30108163

https://www.ncbi.nlm.nih.gov/pubmed/30244201

https://www.ncbi.nlm.nih.gov/pmc/articles/PMC3945587/

https://www.ncbi.nlm.nih.gov/books/NBK499830/

https://www.ncbi.nlm.nih.gov/pmc/articles/PMC6371871/

https://www.ncbi.nlm.nih.gov/books/NBK537084/

https://www.ncbi.nlm.nih.gov/books/NBK537084/

https://www.ncbi.nlm.nih.gov/pmc/articles/PMC3564212/

https://www.ncbi.nlm.nih.gov/pmc/articles/PMC4822166/

https://www.ncbi.nlm.nih.gov/pmc/articles/PMC4822166/

https://www.ncbi.nlm.nih.gov/pmc/articles/PMC6024699/

https://www.ncbi.nlm.nih.gov/pmc/articles/PMC5598025/

Manufactured by Amazon.ca
Bolton, ON

39352232R00069